D0991694

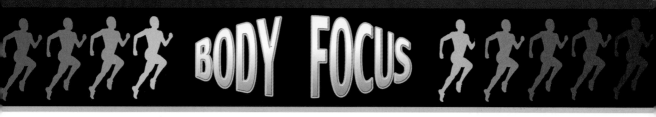

The Immune System

Injury, Illness and Health

Carol Ballard

Heinemann Library
Chicago, Illinois

Design: Jo Hinton-Malivoire and AMR
Illustrations: Art Construction

Originated by Blenheim Colour Ltd
Printed in China by Wing King Tong

07 06 05 04
10 9 8 7 6 5 4 3 2

Library of Congress Cataloging-in-Publication Data
Ballard, Carol.
   The immune system / Carol Ballard.
      v. cm. -- (Body focus)
Includes bibliographical references and index.
Contents: Introduction to the immune system -- Things to defend against -- Health and hygiene -- General defense -- Inflammatory response -- Phagocytosis -- Lymphatic system.
   ISBN: 1-40340-751-7 (HC), 1-40343-299-6 (Pbk.)
   1. Immune system--Juvenile literature. [1. Immune system.] I. Title. II. Series.
   QR181.8 .B355 2003
   616.07'9--dc21

                    2002152973

Acknowledgments
The author and publisher are grateful to the following for permission to reproduce copyright material:
p. 6 Creatas; p. 8 SPL/Science Pictures Ltd; p. 9 SPL/Matt Meadows, Peter Arnold Inc; p. 10 SPL/Susumu Nishinaga; pp. 7, 13 SPL/Dr P. Marazzi; p. 15 SPL/Dr Kari Lounatmaa; p. 18 SPL/Mark Clarke; p. 20 SPL/Secchj Loecadle/ CNRI; p. 21 SPL/Alfred Pasieka; pp. 22 (left), 22 (right) SPL/Dr Andrejs Liepjns; p. 26 SPL/National Library of Medicine; p. 27 SPL/Aaron Haupt; p. 29 SPL/James Holmes, Celltec Ltd; p. 30 SPL/Professor S. Cinti/CNRI; p. 32 SPL/Cordelia Molloy; p. 33 SPL/James King Holmes; pp. 34, 42 SPL/CNRI; p. 35 Arena/PAL; p. 36 Corbis/Bettman; p. 37 Cornell University; p. 38 SPL/Scott Camazine/ CDC; p. 40 SPL/Ed Young; p. 41 Corbis/Annie Griffiths Bell; p. 43 Alamy.

The cover image of a transmission electron micrograph of the AIDS virus appears courtesy of Science Photo Library/Chris Bjonberg.

The publisher would like to thank David Wright and Kelley Staley for their assistance with the preparation of this book.

Every effort has been made to contact copyright holders of any material reproduced in this book. Any omissions will be rectified in subsequent printings if notice is given to the publisher.

Some words are shown in bold, **like this.** You can find out what they mean by looking in the glossary.

CONTENTS

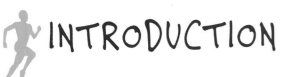# INTRODUCTION

The immune system is the body's defense mechanism against disease. It involves a variety of cells, tissues, and organs, all of which work together in different ways to keep the body free from illness and disease. Some mechanisms are nonspecific. They respond in the same way to any potential problem. Other mechanisms are very specific, responding to only a single stimulus.

Skin

The body is completely covered by skin. This provides the body's first means of defense. Skin forms a barrier between the tissues and the air in the environment. It prevents dirt and **microbes** from entering the body.

Blood

The blood plays an important part in defending the body. It is an efficient transport system, carrying essential chemicals and cells to sites of injury and removing dead cells and other debris. **Platelets** help to form scabs over wounds, keeping infection out and allowing healing to take place. White blood cells act in a variety of ways to prevent infections and diseases.

Lymphatic system

The **lymphatic system** is a network of drainage tubes and related tissues and organs. A watery fluid called **lymph** flows around the body through this network. White blood cells are produced in the red **bone marrow,** and some travel to lymphoid tissue to mature. Many white blood cells are stored in **lymph nodes** to be released into the bloodstream when they are needed. Some microbes can be trapped in lymph nodes for destruction by white blood cells.

Doctors use methods such as **vaccination** to stimulate the immune system and prevent disease.

This diagram shows the lymphatic system, the network of channels through which lymph flows around the body. The lymph nodes, **spleen,** and **thymus** are also part of the system.

Blood cells play an important part in defending the body. Different blood cells respond in different ways. Your skin provides an effective barrier, stopping microbes from entering the body.

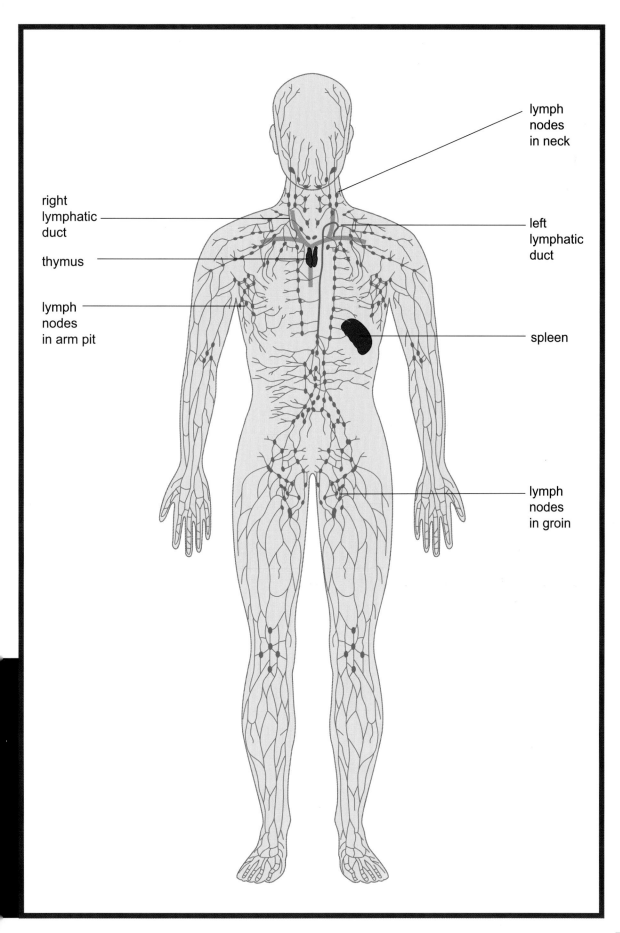

lymph
nodes
in neck

right
lymphatic
duct

left
lymphatic
duct

thymus

lymph
nodes
in arm pit

spleen

lymph
nodes
in groin

DEFENSE AGAINST WHAT?

The body is exposed to many different chemicals, foreign materials, and **microbes** every day. The majority do not pose any threat at all, but some could cause damage and illness. The body must defend itself against these. It must also recognize and defend itself against any abnormal changes that occur within it.

Foreign objects

The inside of the body needs to be kept as clean as possible. So it is important that dust, dirt, and other foreign objects be prevented from entering it.

Toxins

Toxins are poisonous chemicals made by other animals, plants, or **microorganisms.** Some cause only a small reaction, such as a rash after touching poison ivy, or a sore red area after an insect bite. The body can successfully defend itself against such toxins, and little damage occurs. Some toxins, such as those found in snake venom, are much more dangerous and can be deadly, because the body has no adequate defense against them.

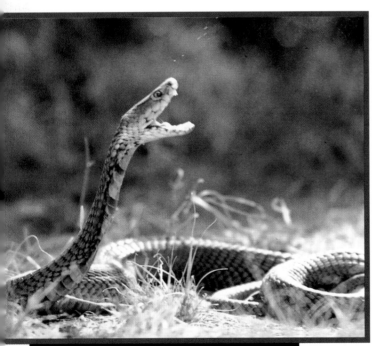

The body has mechanisms to defend itself against toxins. Some, such as that found in this snake's venom, are just too powerful and can be deadly.

Chemicals and poisons

Many everyday chemicals, such as bleach and weedkillers, are potentially dangerous if misused. The body can defend itself against some but not all of these. Your best protection is to make sure you do not unnecessarily expose yourself to any chemicals and always carefully follow all the instructions for proper use.

Bacteria

Bacteria are tiny microbes. They are so tiny, you cannot see them without a microscope. There are many different types of bacteria. Some are entirely harmless, and some, such as the bacteria found in the large **intestine**, are actively useful. However, some bacteria can cause serious illnesses, such as *Escherichia coli* (*E.coli*), which causes serious food poisoning, and *Mycobacterium tuberculosis*, which causes a lung disease known as tuberculosis (TB).

Bacterial infections can occur by eating infected food, inhaling bacteria, having contact with another infected person, and exposing a wound to bacteria in the air.

Viruses

Viruses are much smaller than bacteria and can pass through filters that bacteria cannot. They are transmitted in the same ways as bacteria are and cause many common diseases, such as influenza (flu), chicken pox, and the common cold.

Parasites

Some organisms are parasitic. This means they live inside a host body and get their nourishment from it. Some may eventually kill their host. Some parasites, such as tapeworms, can enter the body by way of food, particularly through meat that is not fully cooked. Others, such as the plasmodium that causes malaria, may be passed to humans by mosquitoes.

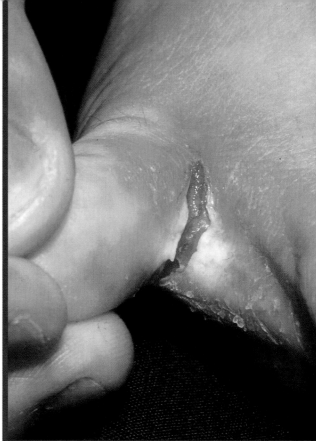

Athlete's foot is caused by a fungus that grows on the dead skin of the feet.

Abnormal body tissues

The body is made up of trillions and trillions of cells. These continuously grow, divide, die, and are replaced by new cells. For the majority of the time, this cycle continues perfectly. Very, very occasionally, a change may occur in a cell or group of cells that makes it grow or divide more rapidly than usual. These changes can lead to the growth of a tumor. If the body recognizes these changes, it can stop the tumor from developing by destroying the abnormal cells.

Fungi

Fungi are microbes that are important to humans. Yeast makes bread rise and ferments alcohol to make wine and beer. Mushrooms are ingredients used in many recipes around the world. However, some fungi can cause diseases. Athlete's foot is an infection caused by a fungus called *Trichophyton*, which lives and grows on the dead skin of the feet. Ringworm is caused by a different fungus, *Microsporum*, that grows in a ring (usually on the head), causing red, itchy patches. Fungal infections are generally passed from person to person by direct contact or by contact with contaminated items, such as towels.

Many infections can easily spread from one person to another. It makes sense to protect yourself from catching an infection and to avoid passing an infection on to others.

Keeping skin, hair, teeth, and nails clean should be a natural part of everybody's daily routine. It prevents a buildup of **microbes** and reduces the chances of infections.

Pimples

Pimples can be a real nuisance, especially when you are a teenager. They often occur as a result of the overproduction of oil by the skin. The excess oil blocks the pores, and **bacteria** build up and feed off the oil. Washing the skin regularly helps to remove the excess oil and the bacteria. Some people find cleansing lotions useful, and in severe cases, doctors may prescribe **antibiotic** creams.

Clean hands

Your hands come in contact with many things every day. As a result, dirt and microbes collect on your skin. It is important to wash your hands thoroughly before you prepare food to avoid contaminating the food. The places where food is stored and prepared also need to be kept clean, along with any utensils. Before you eat, you should wash your hands to avoid eating any dirt or microbes along with the food.

It is very important that you wash your hands after using the toilet, too. Human waste is full of microbes, and these can easily be transferred onto your hands. Washing removes the microbes, which prevents contamination of other surfaces and reduces the risk of making yourself and others ill.

The bacteria growing in this dish came from a person's unwashed hands.

Coughing and sneezing

Viruses, such as those that cause the common cold and influenza (flu), can be passed from one person to another by droplet infection. When you cough or sneeze, droplets of moisture that contain virus particles are forced out of your mouth and nose and into the air around you. Sneezing into a handkerchief and putting a hand in front of your mouth when you cough ensures that the droplets are trapped and disposed of and not left suspended in the air for someone else to breathe in.

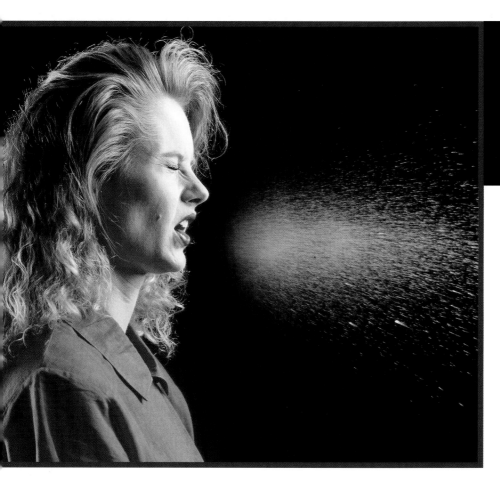

When you sneeze, droplets of moisture are forced out of your nose and into the air.

Spitting

Although most people are probably familiar with the image of baseball players spitting to clear their mouths, spitting excess saliva out of the mouth is less common now than it used to be. It really is something you should try to never do, because it is an easy way to spread germs.

GENERAL DEFENSE

Some of the things that the body needs to defend itself against are quite general. The body does not need to recognize exactly what it is protecting itself from. It just needs to mount a simple defense. There are several efficient mechanisms for doing this.

The air that you breathe in contains dust, dirt, and **microbes.** Ideally, none of these should be allowed to enter your lungs. The inside surfaces of your nose and windpipe are covered with a **membrane** that produces sticky **mucus.** The tiny particles get trapped in the mucus. Fine hairs sweep the mucus away from the lungs, keeping them clean and free from dirt.

Eye protection

Dust and dirt can make your eyes itchy and damage the delicate surfaces. Eyelashes act as filters, keeping many particles away from the surfaces of the eyes. Tears wash over the eyes to clean them. Tears also contain an **enzyme** called lysozyme, which destroys **bacteria.**

Saliva in your mouth washes over your teeth to clean them. It also prevents microbes from growing inside your mouth.

This photograph is a colored scan from an electron micrograph. It shows the tiny hairs of the nose.

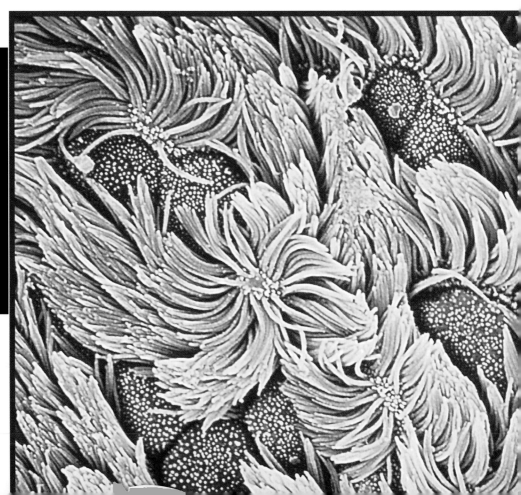

Stomach

The stomach can usually deal effectively with any microbes that enter it. The digestive juices inside the stomach are extremely acidic and will kill most microbes. If toxins enter the stomach, you may vomit to expel them from your body. Toxins and microbes that get past the stomach defenses travel on through the digestive system. If they irritate the lining of the **intestines**, the muscles in the intestinal walls contract strongly. You then suffer from diarrhea, as the microbes are rapidly expelled from the body along with normal digestive waste.

Sebum

The skin forms a barrier between the body tissues and the air around it. Glands in the skin produce an oily substance called sebum, which forms a protective film on top of the skin. Sebum can prevent some bacteria and fungi from growing. The skin is also slightly acidic, and this, too, helps prevent microbe growth. Sweat helps wash microbes from the skin, and it also contains lysozyme, the same enzyme found in tears.

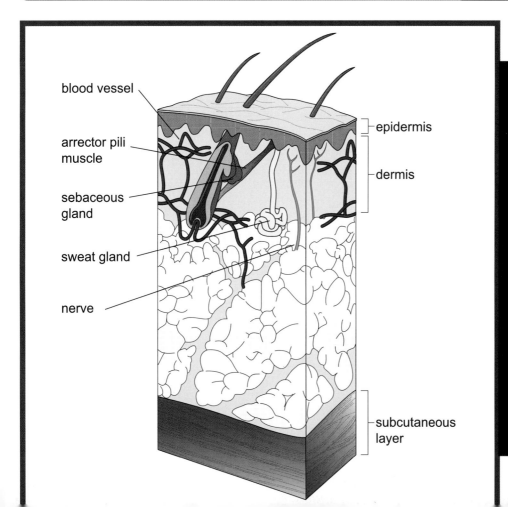

blood vessel

arrector pili muscle

sebaceous gland

sweat gland

nerve

epidermis

dermis

subcutaneous layer

This diagram shows the structure of the skin, the body's natural barrier. The sweat glands produce sweat, and the sebaceous glands produce sebum. Both sweat and sebum help prevent the growth of microbes.

INFLAMMATORY RESPONSE

Damage to body tissues usually results in an **inflammatory response.** This response is nonspecific. The body will react in the same way, whatever the cause of the damage. The skin becomes red and hot, and there is usually swelling and pain.

Causes

Inflammation can be caused by a **viral** or **bacterial** infection; by a physical injury, such as a cut, burn, or bruise; or by an **allergic reaction.** Whatever the cause, the process of inflammation is the same. However, the speed of response may be different. Some responses occur within seconds, others develop slowly over several days.

Steps in the inflammation process

1. Chemical release. When tissue is damaged, a range of different chemicals, including **histamine,** are released. Some of these chemicals affect the local blood vessels; some attract **phagocytes** to the area; and some begin the clotting process to seal the damaged area.

These diagrams show the sequence of events in an inflammatory response:

1. Chemicals are released.
2. Blood vessels widen and their walls become more permeable.
3. Phagocytes arrive.
4. Healing begins.

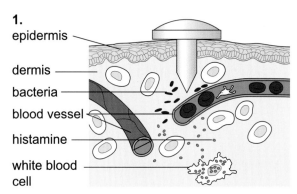

1.
epidermis
dermis
bacteria
blood vessel
histamine
white blood cell

2. swelling

injured cell

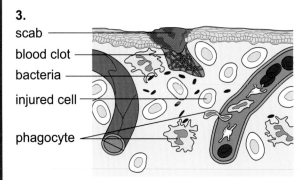

3.
scab
blood clot
bacteria
injured cell
phagocyte

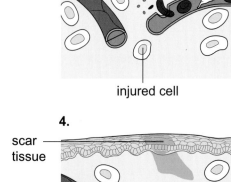

4.
scar tissue

2. Increased blood flow. Blood vessels in the damaged area respond to the chemicals by widening, so more blood can flow through them, speeding up the removal of toxins and dead cells. At the same time, the walls of the blood vessels allow chemicals and specialized blood cells to pass through them into the tissues.

The increased blood flow causes the tissues to become hot and red and may lead to swelling. Pain can be due to damage to nerve fibers, irritation by toxins, or pressure from the swelling.

3. Arrival of phagocytes. Phagocytes move out of the bloodstream, through the blood vessel walls, and into the damaged tissues. They engulf and destroy damaged tissue, worn out blood cells, and **microbes.**

4. Healing. When all the damaged tissue and microbes have been removed, new tissue can begin to grow back into the damaged area. As this healing begins, the phagocytes die and collect together with other debris to form a liquid called pus. This may drain internally or seep out through the skin. If pus cannot drain, an abscess may form.

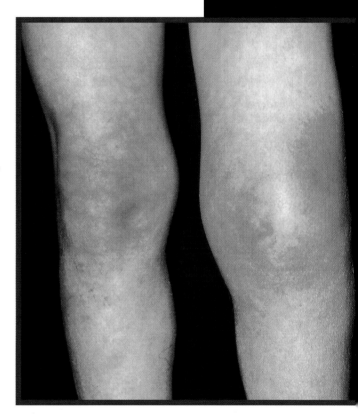

In this photograph, you can see the red, swollen area of inflammation from a wasp sting. It probably also feels hot and painful.

Abscesses

Most abscesses are minor and cause few problems, but others can be more severe and potentially dangerous. The bacterial infection and pus usually cause an area of redness that is hot, swollen, and painful. **Lymph nodes** close to the site of the abscess may also swell as the immune system fights the infection. Some abscesses clear up on their own, but others may need to be treated with **antibiotics** to kill the bacteria. If there is a lot of pus, it may be necessary for a doctor to make a small cut in the skin to allow it to drain. The main danger with an abscess is that it may release harmful bacteria into the bloodstream, and the infection may spread through the body.

PHAGOCYTOSIS

Phagocytosis is the process by which a cell surrounds, engulfs, and destroys other cells, **microbes,** and debris. Its is carried out by specialized white blood cells called **neutrophils** and **macrophages.**

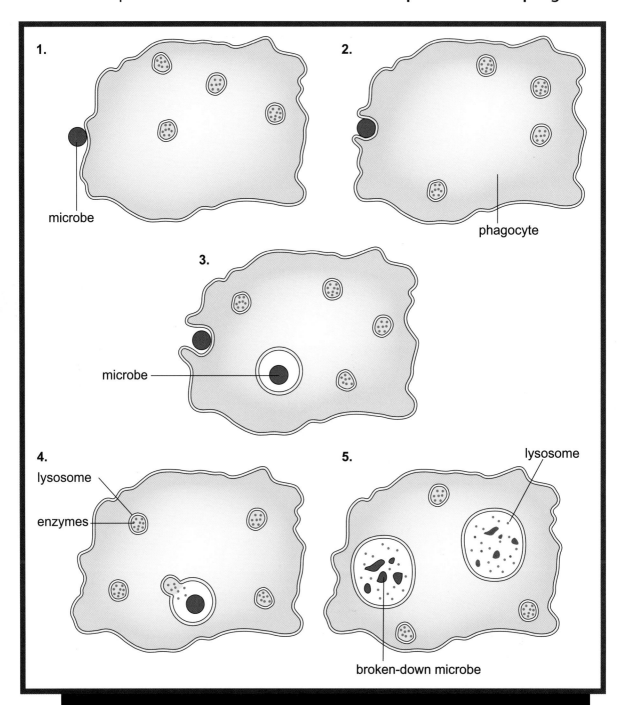

1.

microbe

2.

phagocyte

3.

microbe

4.

lysosome

enzymes

5.

lysosome

broken-down microbe

These diagrams show how a microbe is destroyed by phagocytosis.
1. A phagocyte is attracted to an area of damage by chemicals.
2. The phagocyte attaches itself to a microbe.
3. The phagocyte surrounds and engulfs the microbe.
4. Enzymes from a lysosome break down the microbe.
5. The chemicals from the microbe are emptied outside the phagocyte.

There are five main stages in the process of phagocytosis:

1. Chemical attraction—chemotaxis. **Phagocytes** are attracted to an area of damaged tissue by special chemicals that are released by other white blood cells, damaged tissue cells, and some microbes.

2. Attachment—adherence. The phagocyte attaches itself to the surface of a microbe.

3. Engulfing—ingestion. The cell **membrane** of the phagocyte slowly surrounds the microbe, engulfing it completely. The microbe is sealed inside a small sac of the phagocyte's membrane. This detaches itself from the rest of the membrane and moves further into the phagocyte.

4. Breakdown—digestion. The sac containing the microbe fuses with a baglike structure called a lysosome. This contains **enzymes** that break down every part of the microbe into separate chemicals.

5. Expulsion—exocytosis. Some of the chemicals released by the breakdown of the microbe may be used by the phagocyte. Any unwanted chemicals are emptied outside the phagocyte.

In this photograph taken with an electron micrograph, you can see **bacteria** that have been engulfed by two phagocytes.

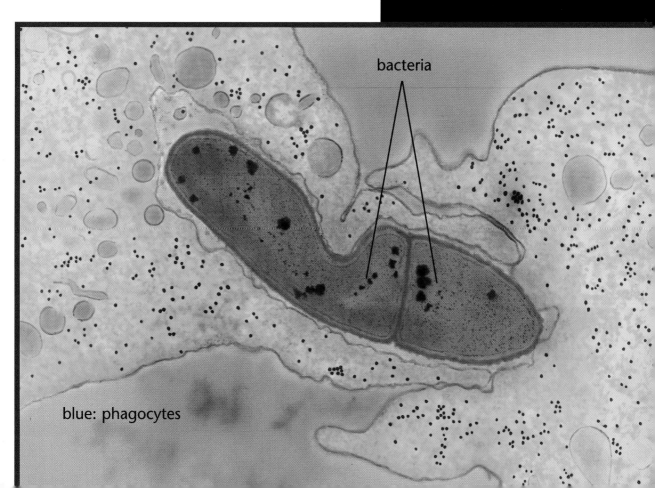

bacteria

blue: phagocytes

LYMPHATIC SYSTEM

The **lymphatic system** consists of a network of drainage tubes: lymphatic vessels, **lymph nodes,** the **spleen,** and the **thymus. Lymph** flows around the body through the lymphatic vessels, removing excess fluid and white blood cells from body tissues.

The spleen

The spleen is about 4.7 inches (12 centimeters) long and lies between the ribs and stomach on the left side of the body. It has a rich supply of blood vessels and lymphatic vessels and plays an important part in filtering the blood. The spleen is also a storage site for blood. It releases blood into the body as needed. An outer capsule encloses two types of tissue, red pulp and white pulp. Red pulp is made up of veins and spaces around them, both filled with blood. White pulp is lymphatic tissue. These tissues are mainly white blood cells arranged around central arteries.

As the spleen filters the blood, dead and abnormal blood cells are removed and recycled. The spleen also removes **microbes** and toxins, and as the white blood cells within the spleen come into contact with these microbes and toxins, a specific immune response may begin.

An injury to the abdomen can rupture the spleen. If this happens, the spleen must be removed right away to prevent massive internal bleeding. In some illnesses, the spleen may become enlarged and may need to be removed. While the spleen is important, a person can live normally without it, because the red **bone marrow** and liver can take over its functions.

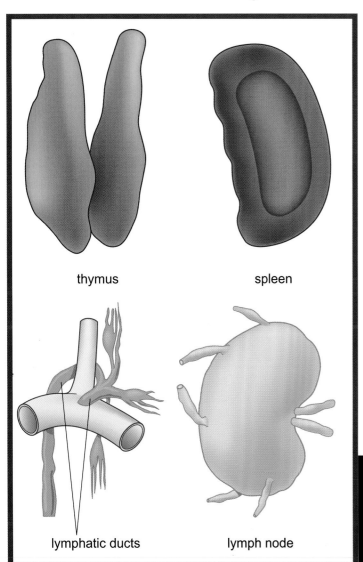

thymus

spleen

lymphatic ducts

lymph node

These diagrams show the thymus, spleen, lymph ducts, and a lymph node.

The thymus gland

The thymus is a mass of lymphoid tissue located in the chest above the heart. It has two lobes joined by connective tissue. It is surrounded by an outer capsule. Each lobe has two areas, the cortex and the medulla. The thymus gland is small. It weighs only about 0.5 oz (15 g) at birth. It enlarges in childhood to reach a maximum size of about 1.2 oz (35 g) in the early teens. It then slowly shrinks and may only weigh 0.1 oz (3 g) in old age. It is most active during childhood, when it is involved in the development of specific immune responses. Some white blood cells travel to the thymus to mature and develop.

Tonsils

The tonsils are small lymphatic nodules inside a capsule. There are three pairs: one pair at the base of the tongue, one pair split at each side of the soft palate (the partition between the nose and mouth), and one pair behind the nose (often called the adenoids). Together, they form a chain of lymphoid tissue at the entrances to the throat to prevent infections from reaching the lungs and digestive system. They contain white blood cells, which destroy invading microbes.

The tonsils themselves often become infected and may be surgically removed. This is a minor procedure, and the patient usually suffers no side effects.

This is a cross section of a lymph node.

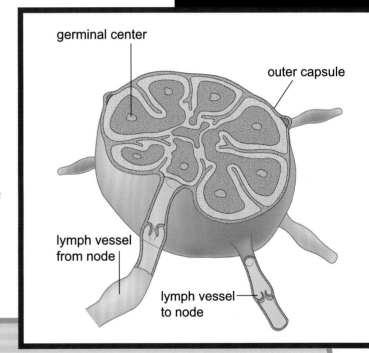

germinal center

outer capsule

lymph vessel from node

lymph vessel to node

Lymph nodes

Lymph nodes are small, beanlike swellings along the lymphatic vessels. They are spread throughout the body, but there are large numbers of them in the armpits, groin, and neck. They have an outer capsule, with fingerlike branches of tissue inside that divide them into separate spaces (similar to the segments of an orange). At the heart of each segment is the germinal center, where some white blood cells are produced.

Lymph nodes store white blood cells, which they release into the lymphatic vessels when they are needed. From there, the cells can move into the bloodstream. Lymph nodes also trap microbes for destruction by the white blood cells.

SPECIFIC IMMUNITY

In addition to having general forms of defense, the body can mount a range of highly effective responses against specific **microbes** and other invading agents. Such a response is specific to that stimulus alone and will not offer any protection against a different stimulus.

Specific immunity is the name given to the body's response to a specific stimulus. A stimulus that makes the body respond is called an **antigen.** There are two important differences between specific immunity and general defense mechanisms:

- Specific immunity protects against one antigen only, whereas general defense mechanisms protect the body from a whole range of invading agents.
- Specific immunity involves a memory function, so a second exposure to the antigen leads to a very strong and rapid response. General defense mechanisms do not involve a memory function.

Specific immunity may be innate (see box below) or acquired.

Innate immunity
Innate immunity means immunity that you are born with. Some species are immune to diseases that affect other species. For example, humans are immune to canine distemper, which affects dogs. Within a species, some individuals are immune to diseases that affect other individuals. If one child in a family catches chicken pox, for example, a brother or sister may be exposed to the **virus** but not develop the disease.

This child has chicken pox— but catching it when he is young allows his body to defend itself against chicken pox for the rest of his life.

Acquired immunity

Any immunity that is not present at birth must have been acquired by exposure to a specific antigen. The body responds to the antigen and is then able to store the memory of the antigen.

There are several ways of acquiring immunity:

Active immunity:

- Immunity can be acquired by natural exposure to the antigen during the course of a disease. This can provide lifelong immunity. Having chicken pox as a child, for example, means that you are extremely unlikely to suffer from it a second time.
- Immunity can also be acquired by artificial exposure to the antigen. This can be achieved by injection of dead or weakened antigens through **vaccination**. These stimulate the body to mount a specific immune response. Vaccines can provide lifelong protection, but some, such as tetanus, require repeated injections called boosters every few years.

Passive immunity:

- Immunity can be acquired naturally from outside the body. Immunity can pass from a mother to her baby during pregnancy or breast-feeding. This provides protection for several months while the baby's own immune system is developing.
- Immunity can be acquired by injecting **serum** from an immune person into another individual. This provides protection for a short period of weeks or months.

Exercise and immunity

Research has shown that there may be a link between exercise and immunity. Scientists think that light to moderate exercise can boost the immune system, but that high-intensity exercise can actually have a negative effect on health. Try not to train too hard when there is a high risk of infection, such as in winter when there are a lot of coughs and colds around. It is also a good idea to reduce the intensity of exercise when you are under extra physical or emotional stress.

This table summarizes the different ways of acquiring immunity.

Acquired immunity	Active	Passive
natural	exposure to antigen during the course of a disease	from mother to baby during pregnancy or breast-feeding
artificial	injection of dead or weakened antigen	injection of immune serum

WHITE BLOOD CELLS

The body's defenses against invading **microbes** and abnormal cells are carried out by white blood cells. There are several types of white blood cells, each specialized to do its own specific job. Together, white blood cells are known as leukocytes.

All white blood cells originate from **stem cells** in the red **bone marrow.** As these divide, more cells are produced, and these, in turn, divide to produce even more cells. The process is like a waterfall, with small changes taking place at each stage so that, from one original stem cell, a whole range of highly specialized cells are produced.

The origination of white blood cells:

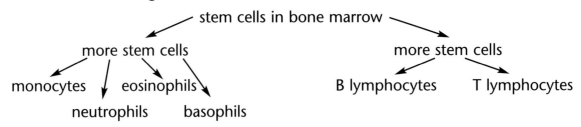

stem cells in bone marrow

more stem cells

monocytes   eosinophils
      neutrophils   basophils

more stem cells

B lymphocytes   T lymphocytes

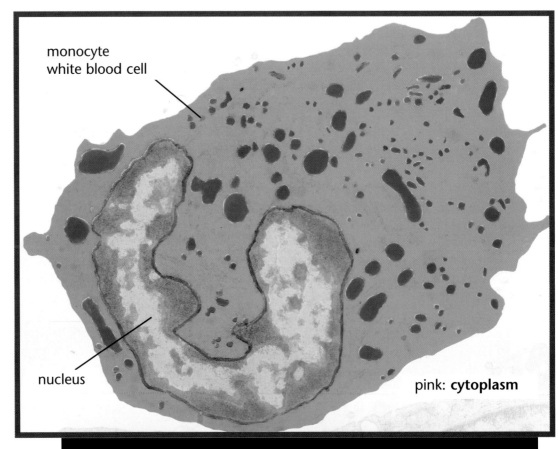

monocyte
white blood cell

nucleus

pink: **cytoplasm**

This photograph has been taken using a microscope. The white blood cell has been stained with chemicals so that the internal structures can be seen.

Types of white blood cells

Cells from stem cells are produced in the bone marrow. Some are fully matured when they leave. **Neutrophils** are specialized **phagocytes** involved in general defense mechanisms, engulfing and destroying microbes and other cells. Monocytes are types of phagocytes, too. They move into body tissues and enlarge to become wandering **macrophages**. These also engulf and destroy microbes and dead tissue cells. Eosinophils and basophils are involved in **allergic reactions** and **inflammatory responses**.

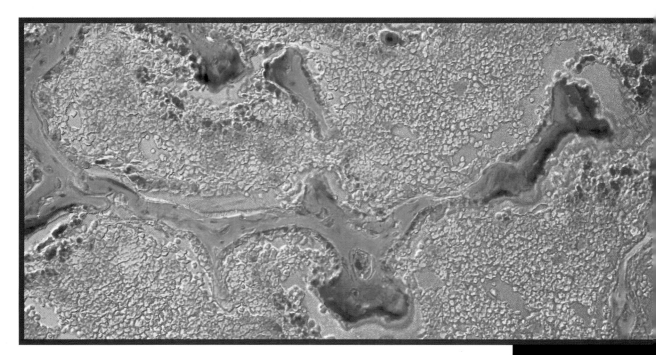

This photograph is of red marrow inside a bone. It is from this tissue that white blood cells develop.

Lymphocytes

Some cells from stem cells leave the bone marrow before they are fully mature. These cells develop into **lymphocytes** at other places in the body. There are two main groups of lymphocytes:

- B lymphocytes. These leave the bone marrow and travel to lymphoid tissues, such as the **spleen** and **lymph nodes.** They move into the lymphoid tissue, and more B lymphocytes are produced in these tissues without the involvement of the bone marrow. B lymphocytes are involved in specific immune responses. They produce chemical responses to specific **antigens.**

- T lymphocytes. These also leave the bone marrow and travel straight to the **thymus,** where they develop fully. They are involved in specific immune responses, regulating the actions of B lymphocytes and other cells. Some T lymphocytes can kill microbes and other cells.

CELL-MEDIATED IMMUNITY

The body's response to a specific **antigen** consists of several different processes and pathways. These are interlinked but can be thought of in two main categories: responses by specific cells, called cell-mediated immunity, and responses involving the release of chemicals known as **antibodies.** Many antigens cause both types of responses.

T-cells

T **lymphocytes,** or T-cells, are responsible for cell-mediated immunity. Their responses involve direct contact between the T-cell and the antigen, and they always involve attacking and killing cells. Cell-mediated responses occur when T-cells are stimulated by parasites, fungi, **bacteria,** and **viruses.** They also occur when T-cells recognize abnormal body cells, such as cancer cells and tissue transplant cells.

There are three main types of T-cells:
- Helper T-cells. These help activate B lymphocytes (B-cells) and **macrophages.** They also help other T-cells.
- Suppressor T-cells. These help reduce the responses of other cells, preventing the immune system from overreacting and damaging the body itself.
- Killer T-cells. These have specific receptors for antigens. When they come into direct contact with a **microbe** or other abnormal cell, they release chemicals onto its surface that makes the cell leak, which destroys it.

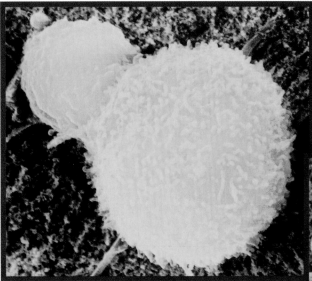

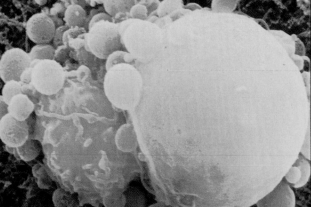

The top electron micrograph shows a large cancer cell and a smaller killer T-cell. In the bottom picture, you can see that the cancer cell is beginning to leak as chemicals from the T-cells attack its **membrane.**

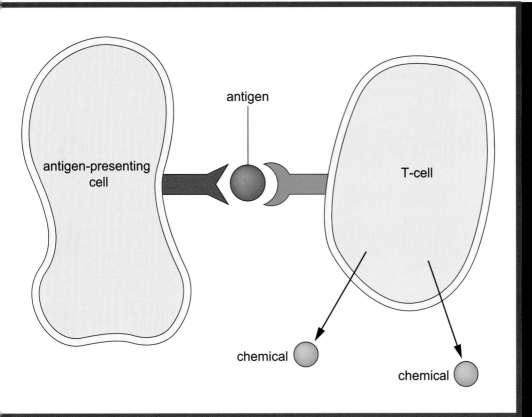

antigen

antigen-presenting cell

T-cell

chemical

chemical

In cell-mediated immunity, an antigen is picked up by an antigen-presenting cell and displayed for a T-cell to identify as foreign. The T-cell then attacks and produces chemicals that alert other cells in the immune system that there is an infection.

Balancing act

The helper cells and suppressor cells have a finely tuned control over the system, balancing each other and making sure that exactly the right level of immune response is generated.

There are millions of different T-cells, each programmed to respond to one specific antigen. When a T-cell meets the antigen it is programmed to recognize, it divides over and over to produce a clone of identical T-cells, all programmed to recognize the antigen. Some of these become helper cells, some become suppressor cells, and others become killer cells. The killer cells kill the cells carrying the antigen. Once all the cells are killed, the suppressor cells take over and the immune response fades away. Any T-cells from the clone that are left become memory cells. If the same antigen invades the body again, thousands of memory cells are ready to mount an immediate attack. At this point, there are more memory cells and the response is much faster and stronger than it was the first time the antigen was encountered.

Cancer cells
Cancer cells have special antigens on their surfaces that are not on the surfaces of normal cells. Some T-cells are programmed to recognize these antigens and destroy the cells swiftly, thus preventing a tumor from growing and developing.

ANTIBODIES AND IMMUNITY

B **lymphocytes** (B-cells) respond to **antigens** by releasing chemicals called **antibodies,** which circulate in the **lymph** and blood. Each antibody is specific to one particular antigen. The antibody and antigen become attached to each other when they meet.

There are millions of different B lymphocytes. Each is programmed to respond to one specific antigen by producing and releasing one specific type of antibody.

A B-cell becomes activated when it comes into contact with the antigen it is programmed to respond to. It divides again and again, producing a clone of identical B-cells. Each cell produces identical antibody molecules and releases them into the blood and **lymph.**

This diagram shows how antibodies and antigens fit together, making it easier for phagocytes to destroy the antigen.

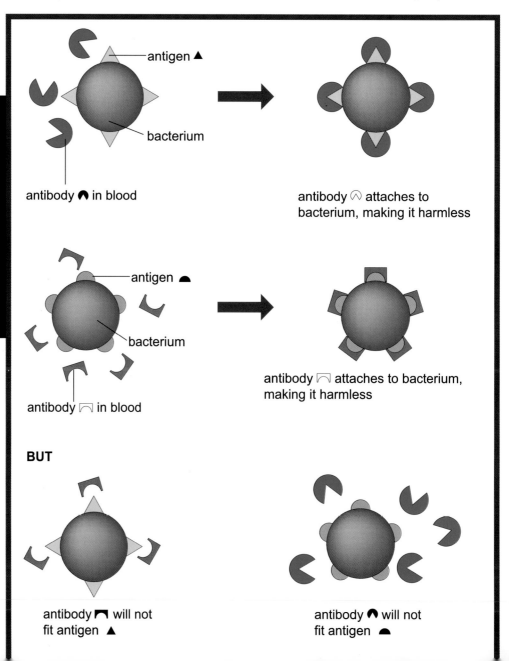

antigen ▲

bacterium

antibody ⌒ in blood

antibody ⌒ attaches to bacterium, making it harmless

antigen ◖

bacterium

antibody ⌒ in blood

antibody ⌒ attaches to bacterium, making it harmless

BUT

antibody ⌒ will not fit antigen ▲

antibody ⌒ will not fit antigen ◖

When antibody and antigen combine

Each antibody molecule can combine with the specific antigen. They fit together the way a lock and key fit together. The main effect of their coming together is that it becomes easier for **phagocytes** to engulf and destroy the antigen. Other things can also happen when the antigen and antibody combine:

- Some **bacterial** toxins are neutralized so they cannot do any further damage.
- Some **viruses** are made harmless by being prevented from attaching to body cells.
- Some bacteria are prevented from moving.
- Some **microbes** are forced to clump together.

Unlike T lymphocytes (T-cells), the B-cells stay in their places in the lymphoid tissue. All that circulate are the antibody molecules. When the response is over, any B-cells from the clone that remain become memory cells, able to mount a swift and strong attack if the body is exposed to that same antigen again.

These diagrams show how the protein chains are arranged in the different types of Ig molecule.

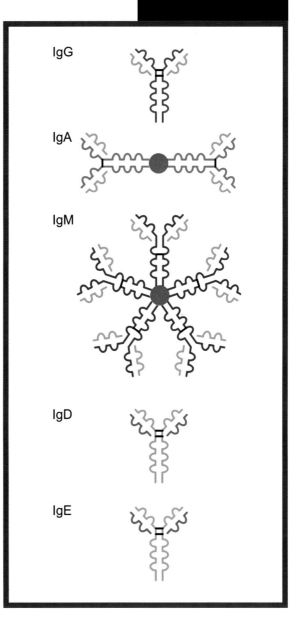

IgG

IgA

IgM

IgD

IgE

What are antibodies?

Antibodies are complex **protein** molecules called immunoglobulins (Ig). There are five main types: IgA, IgD, IgE, IgG, and IgM. Each molecule is made up of protein chains, both heavy and light. The chains are arranged differently in different types of Ig molecules. Some parts of the chains are constant and are the same for all Ig molecules. Other parts of the chains are variable, allowing each Ig molecule to be specific for one specific antigen.

Vaccination is a way of providing protection against potentially dangerous diseases. This is done by exposing the immune system to a small amount of disease material that has been made harmless. Massive vaccination programs around the world have almost eliminated many diseases. However, there are still arguments about how safe some vaccinations are.

The first vaccination

The first recorded vaccination was carried out by Dr. Edward Jenner in England in 1796. At that time, smallpox was a deadly disease that killed many people every year. Cowpox was a similar disease that affected cows. Humans could catch cowpox, too, but it was much less serious than smallpox. Jenner noticed that milkmaids who caught cowpox did not catch smallpox.

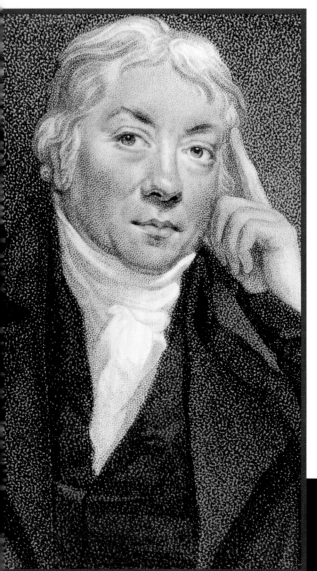

Jenner decided to try an experiment. He infected a young boy with cowpox and waited for him to fully recover. Then, Jenner infected the boy with deadly smallpox and waited to see what would happen. He hoped that the previous exposure to cowpox would protect the boy and save him from developing smallpox. Jenner was right. The boy stayed well.

Other doctors and scientists were not convinced at first. Jenner carried out more experiments and published his results. His process became known as vaccination, taken from the Latin word for a cow, *vacca*. Eventually, Jenner's ideas became accepted, and vaccination became widespread. Vaccination against smallpox has been very successful, and today smallpox is found only in freezers in secure biological laboratories.

Edward Jenner developed the technique of vaccination against smallpox.

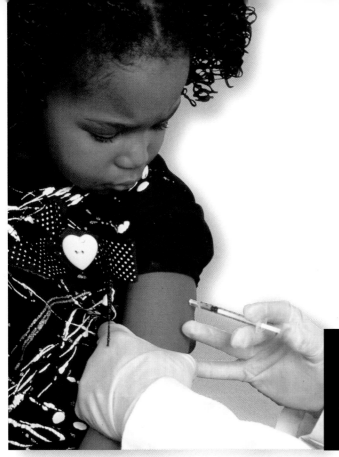

Developing vaccines

Following Jenner's work on smallpox, scientists began to develop vaccines for other diseases. The most well-known of these are Louis Pasteur's vaccine for rabies, discovered in the 1880s, and Jonas Salk's vaccine for poliomyelitis, which came into general use in the early 1950s.

This child is being vaccinated to protect her from serious childhood diseases.

Vaccination programs

Most countries now run comprehensive vaccination programs, which children start when they are very young. Many people are routinely vaccinated against diseases such as tuberculosis, diphtheria, and poliomyelitis. When people travel abroad, they often have vaccinations against diseases they may not encounter in their own country, such as malaria and yellow fever.

Safety

There are still a lot of arguments about the safety of some vaccinations. In recent years, a combined vaccine for mumps, measles, and rubella has become available. Some doctors think that there might be a connection between this vaccine and certain conditions, including autism and some bowel diseases. Some parents are happy to have their children vaccinated, some choose not to vaccinate their children at all, and others choose to get the three vaccines separately. There are arguments for and against each course of action.

How do vaccines work?

When you are vaccinated, you are injected with a small amount of dead or weakened **microbe** material. Your immune system responds to this as if it were real, live material. T-cells and B-cells become activated, **antibodies** are produced, and a full specific immune response is launched. Memory cells remain afterward, and as a result, if live microbes invade your body in the future, the memory cells are ready to mount a swift and strong attack. This prevents you from suffering from the illness.

MONOCLONAL ANTIBODIES

Antibodies are **proteins** that are produced by B **lymphocytes** in response to specific **antigens.** Scientists have developed ways of producing large amounts of identical antibodies that can be used for a variety of purposes. These are called monoclonal antibodies.

Developing the technique

In 1975 two scientists, Georges Kohler and Cesar Milstein, produced the first monoclonal antibodies and were awarded a Nobel Prize for their work. They injected an antigen into a mouse and then removed activated lymphocytes from the mouse's **spleen.** In their laboratory, they fused an activated lymphocyte with a tumor cell, thus producing a new type of cell called a hybridoma. This new cell divided again and again, producing a clone of identical cells. Each cell produced identical antibodies to the antigen they had originally injected into the mouse. The scientists' technique gave them an unlimited supply of identical **antibody** molecules. Because all the antibodies came from one clone, they were called monoclonal antibodies.

This diagram shows the stages in the production of monoclonal antibodies.
1. A mouse is injected with the antigen.
2. The mouse's immune system is stimulated, and lymphocytes are activated.
3. Active lymphocytes are collected and fused with a tumor cell to make hybridoma.
4. A tumor cell is used because it is able to divide many times.
5. Hybridoma cells divide many times to make clones of identical cells.
6. Clone cells produce antibodies.
7. Monoclonal antibodies are isolated for cultivation.

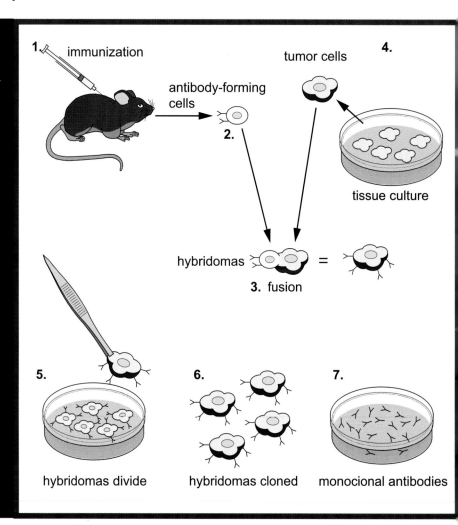

1. immunization
tumor cells
4.
antibody-forming cells
2.
tissue culture
hybridomas =
3. fusion
5. hybridomas divide
6. hybridomas cloned
7. monocional antibodies

Monoclonal antibodies can be used for a variety of things:

- reducing **rejection** of tissue transplants
- treatment of some inflammatory diseases
- prevention of clogged arteries in patients with heart disease.

Rejection of tissue transplants

The United States government approved the use of a monoclonal antibody in kidney transplant patients in 1986. This antibody attacks the T lymphocytes (T-cells) that cause tissue rejection. Doctors have found that patients who are given the monoclonal antibody are significantly less likely to reject the transplanted kidney than patients given more conventional drug treatments.

Other uses

Some other applications of monoclonal antibodies are in cancer treatment. Antibodies can be made to be specific to antigens found on the surface of cancer cells. If an anticancer drug is attached to the antibodies, the antibodies will deliver the drug straight to the cancer cells without causing damage to any other cells and tissues. A special tracer could also be linked to cancer-specific antibodies and be used to find out the precise location of cancer cells.

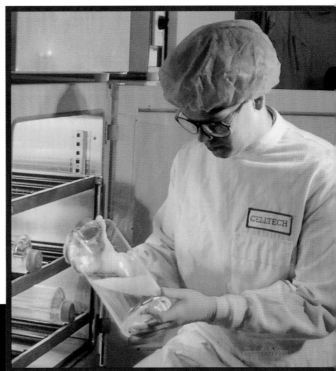

This scientist is isolating cells for use in monoclonal antibody production.

Problems with monoclonal antibodies

There are some problems in the production and use of monoclonal antibodies. The human immune system can recognize the mouse material within the monoclonal antibodies and quickly mounts an immune response to destroy them. Also, people are increasingly uncomfortable with the use of animals in science. However, without mice, scientists have no simple way of producing the initial active lymphocytes needed. It is possible to use humans instead, but few people would be happy with this idea.

An **allergy** is sensitivity to something that most people do not react to. The substance that causes the allergy is called an allergen. Allergies to many everyday substances such as pollen, insect stings, animal fur, and house dust mites are common. Some **allergic reactions** can be very quick, developing almost immediately, while other allergic reactions can take hours or days to develop.

Immediate allergic reaction

This type of reaction develops within minutes of exposure to the allergen. B **lymphocytes** (B-cells) respond to the allergen by producing extra IgE **antibodies.** These bind to the surface of some white blood cells. The allergen particles bind to the IgE antibodies, and the white blood cells release **histamine** and other chemicals. These start an **inflammatory response** and may also cause muscle contractions in the airways and increased production of **mucus.** The person may suffer from inflammation and may have difficulty breathing and a runny nose.

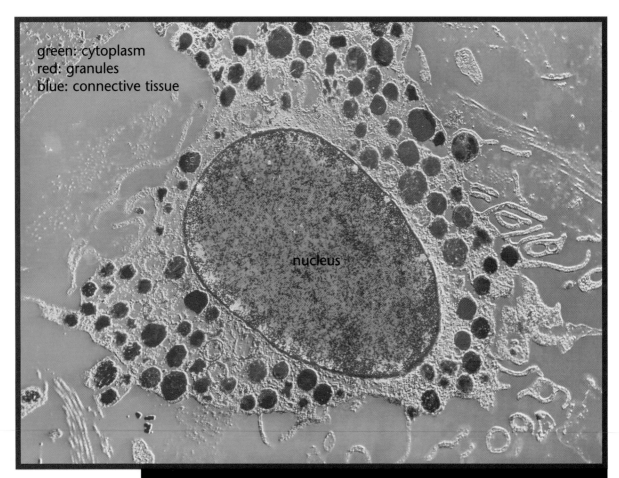

green: cytoplasm
red: granules
blue: connective tissue

nucleus

This photomicrograph shows a white blood cell with granules that contain histamine, serotonin, and herapin.

Anaphylactic shock

Severe allergic reactions are known as **anaphylactic shock.** Such reactions are life-threatening and must be treated as quickly as possible. People who know they are at risk for anaphylactic shock usually carry a small device called an EpiPen. The device contains a simple mechanism that allows the person to inject a dose of epinephrine into a muscle. Epinephrine makes breathing easier and helps control the heartbeat. A medical bracelet is often also worn, with details of the person's condition, so other people know what treatment should be given.

Anaphylactic shock is not common, but some allergens are known to provoke very swift and severe reactions. Wasp and bee stings can provoke anaphylactic shock in sensitized people, and an increasing number of people are experiencing severe allergic reactions to peanuts.

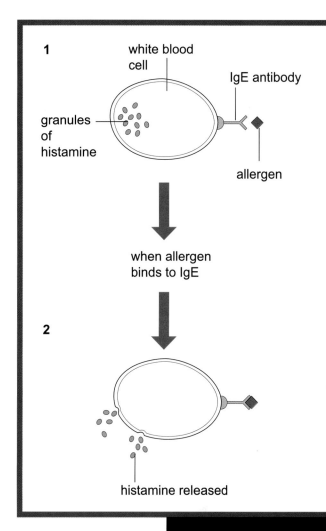

Delayed allergic reaction

In some cases, the allergic reaction does not appear until 12 to 72 hours after exposure to the allergen. This happens when the allergen travels to the **lymph nodes.** T lymphocytes (T-cells) multiply, and some return to the place where the allergen first entered the body. There, they activate **macrophages,** and an inflammatory response begins.

BCG

The BCG blood test for immunity to tuberculosis (TB) is based on this mechanism. A small amount of inactive TB material is pricked into the skin. After a couple of days, the skin is examined. If a red welt appears, it proves that the person is already sensitive to the tuberculosis **bacterium** and does not need to be **vaccinated.** If there is no red welt, the person is not sensitized to the bacterium, and vaccination will give them protection against the disease.

These diagrams show what happens in an immediate allergic reaction.
1. A white blood cell with an attached IgE antibody comes into contact with an allergen.
2. The allergen attaches to the antibody, and the white blood cell releases histamine.

People who suffer from **allergies** need to find a way to cope with their allergy so that it does not interfere with their life too much. Some allergies are easy to identify, and it may be easy to avoid contact with the allergen. Others are harder to identify, and the allergen may be difficult to avoid.

Airborne allergens

Many people suffer from hay fever. This **allergic reaction** is caused by pollen—usually from grass—in the air. In most cases, hay fever lasts just a short time while grass pollen is released. It may be prolonged if the person is allergic to more than one type of pollen. Hay fever involves red, itchy eyes, a runny nose, and excessive sneezing. During the height of the hay fever season, in May and June, weather forecasts often give a pollen index. If you suffer from hay fever, it is a good idea to avoid being outside too much when there is a lot of pollen in the air. Some drugs, including antihistamines, are available to combat hay fever.

Hay fever causes red, itchy eyes, and a runny nose.

Food allergies

Allergies to foods can produce a wide variety of symptoms. However, there is usually a feeling of sickness, followed by vomiting and diarrhea, within hours of eating the food. In severe cases, the lips and tongue may become red and swollen. A skin rash may also appear hours or days later.

Identifying the substance to which a person is allergic is sometimes very simple. For example, if you know that you always feel sick after eating shellfish, the answer is simple: Don't eat shellfish!

Skin allergies

Touching something to which you are allergic will cause an **inflammatory response.** Common allergens are wool, some metals, some plants, adhesive bandages, and chemicals in some soaps. Many adults suffer from dermatitis, and eczema in children is often caused by allergies. The best way to deal with this type of allergy is to avoid all contact with the allergen, if possible. Creams and ointments can often help to make the dry, cracked skin of eczema more bearable.

Testing for allergies

Identifying allergies is not always straightforward, especially if several different allergens are involved. Doctors may perform skin tests by putting a tiny drop of liquid containing an allergen onto the skin and then pricking it into the skin with a fine needle. If the person is allergic to the allergen, a red welt appears on the skin after a few minutes. Many different allergens can be tested at the same time, each at a different place on the skin.

Skin tests can be used to help identify the cause of an allergy.

Food allergies can often be identified by way of an elimination diet. The person is allowed to eat a very simple diet of water, one type of meat, and one vegetable for a few days. Other foods are introduced one at a time. If the person feels better, the allergen has been excluded. If he or she begins to feel ill again, it must be because of one of the foods added back to their diet. It is important that elimination diets are carried out under the supervision of a doctor so that the person can be properly monitored.

AUTOIMMUNITY

Autoimmunity is the name given to any condition where a person's immune system begins to attack his or her own body.

In most people, the immune system only responds to foreign, or non-self, **antigens.** It recognizes the body's own antigens as self and ignores them. If something goes wrong, the immune system begins to recognize the body's own tissues as non-self and mounts an immune response against them.

Recognizing self

While T **lymphocytes** (T-cells) are maturing in the **thymus** gland, they go through a selection process. Those that recognize body tissues as self and do not react will survive. Any that do not recognize self will die. Any that recognize self and react will also die. A similar process of selection of B lymphocytes (B-cells) occurs as they develop in the **bone marrow.**

There are two main causes of autoimmunity:

- If part of the body becomes damaged in some way, antigens that would normally remain hidden may become exposed to the immune system. Because the immune system has not met them before, it cannot recognize them as self, and so it begins to attack them. An example of this is a condition called sympathetic ophthalmia. In this condition, one eye becomes damaged and new antigens are exposed. The immune system attacks these antigens and the other healthy eye, too.
- A random **genetic** change in a B-cell or T-cell may give rise to a clone of lymphocytes that react against the body's own tissue.

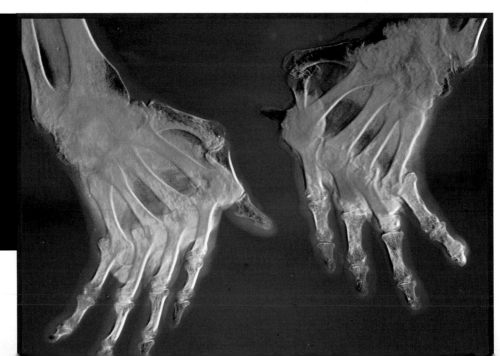

This is an X ray of the hands of a person with rheumatoid arthritis. You can see how the joints are deformed.

Several disease conditions are the result of autoimmunity:

Rheumatoid arthritis

In rheumatoid arthritis, some B-cells change to produce a different form of IgM **antibody,** called rheumatoid factor. This reacts against normal IgG and causes the inflammation of joints. The joints become swollen and painful, eventually becoming deformed and stiff. Treatment with painkillers helps the patient to cope, and a range of drugs, including **steroids,** can often keep the disease under control and prevent some of its crippling effects.

Multiple sclerosis

In multiple sclerosis, the **protein** coverings of nerves become inflamed, damaged, and scarred as a result of action by the body's own immune system. The affected nerves cannot transmit signals to and from the brain properly, and the person's movements are gradually restricted. Although there is some evidence for a **genetic** link, scientists have not proved that it is an inherited condition. A drug, called beta interferon, can slow the progress of the disease in some cases, but it is an expensive treatment and not all patients are able to tolerate the powerful drug.

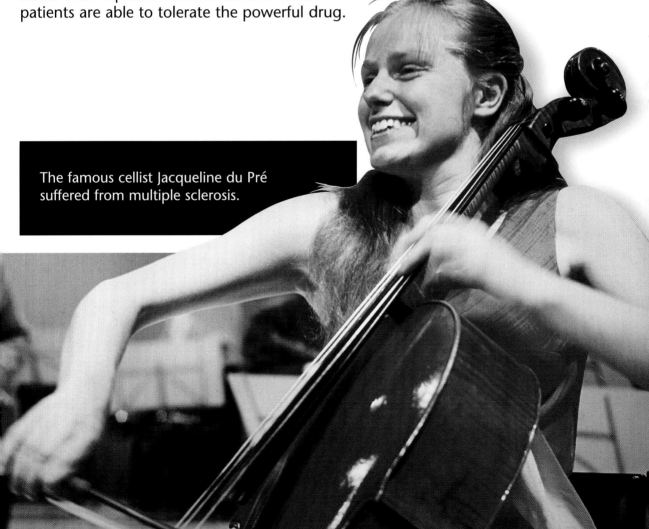

The famous cellist Jacqueline du Pré suffered from multiple sclerosis.

IMMUNODEFICIENCY AND IMMUNOSUPPRESSION

If a person is suffering from an **immunodeficiency** or **immunosuppression,** his or her immune system is unable to respond effectively to **antigens**. This means that he or she is vulnerable to infections and has no way of overcoming them.

Immunodeficiency

Some people are born with an immune system that cannot function. They may have no T or B **lymphocytes** (T- or B-cells). If they have B-cells, they may not be able to produce a full range of **antibodies**.

IgA deficiency

Selective IgA deficiency is a condition in which a person cannot produce IgA antibodies. It is important to protect the body's surfaces that come into contact with its surroundings, such as the mouth and nose, lungs, throat, digestive tract, and eyes. It is mainly IgA that protects these surfaces from infection. People with IgA deficiency, therefore, often suffer from recurrent infections, such as ear infections, sinusitis, and pneumonia. They may have to take **antibiotics** for longer than usual.

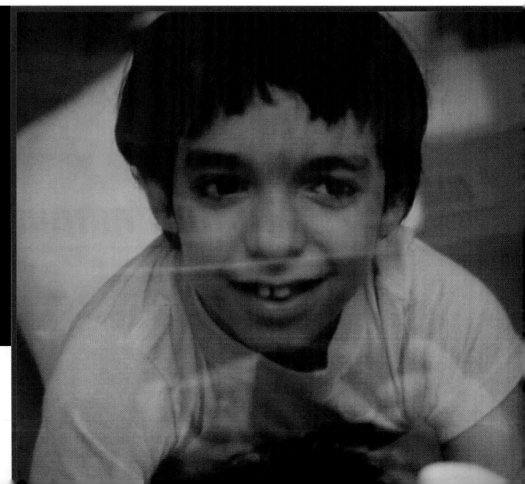

This boy was born with SCID. He has no resistance to infection. He must live enclosed in a sterile plastic bubble until doctors can find a way to get his immune system functioning properly.

Severe combined immunodeficiency syndrome (SCID)

Severe combined immunodeficiency syndrome (SCID) is a very serious, although fortunately rare, inherited condition. Babies born with SCID have no B-cells or T-cells. As a result, they have practically no defense against infection. They often die in early childhood, but **bone marrow** transplants have been found to help some children with SCID.

Immunosuppression

Sometimes, a person's immune system needs to be turned off, or suppressed. Drugs that can do this are called immunosuppressants. They play an important part in helping a person's body accept a tissue transplant, preventing the immune system from recognizing the transplant as non-self and attacking it.

Immunosuppressant drugs have to be used very carefully, however. By turning off a person's immune system, the drugs remove the person's ability to react to an infection. Also, any abnormal cells, such as cancer cells, will not be detected by the immune system while it is turned off, and therefore, will not be attacked.

As people age

Other conditions, such as viral infections, can lead to a reduction in the efficiency of the immune system. As people age, their immune systems slowly become less efficient. T-cells become less responsive to antigens, fewer T-cells respond to infections, and B-cells produce fewer antibodies. Together, these changes mean that as a person ages, he or she is more likely to suffer from infections.

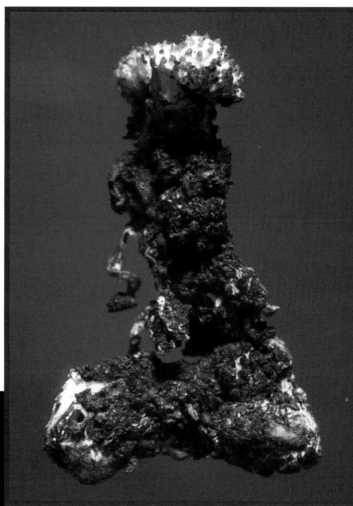

The fungus *Tolypocladium inflatum* produces the immunosuppressant drug cyclosporin.

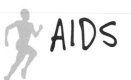 # AIDS

AIDS stands for acquired immune deficiency syndrome and is caused by infection with HIV, or the human **immunodeficiency virus.** Many people with HIV infection do not have AIDS and may show no signs of illness for many years.

There are many myths about HIV and AIDS, and people often feel that they do not want to be around anyone that might have the disease. However, there is no basis for such ideas, because HIV cannot be passed from one person to another by casual contact. The virus is fragile and can only survive outside the body for a short time. It can be killed by disinfectants and by normal washing of dishes and clothes. HIV can only be passed from one person to another by the mixing of body fluids, by sexual contact, or by sharing needles between drug users. Some people with **hemophilia** have been infected with HIV after receiving contaminated blood products, but all blood donations are now screened for HIV in an attempt to prevent this from happening in the future.

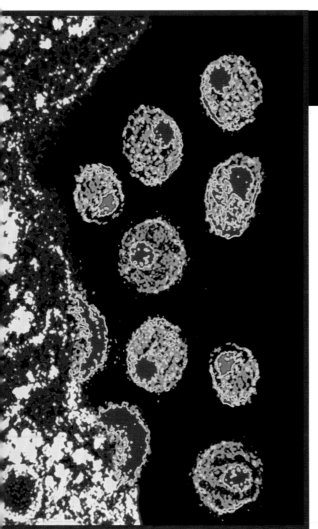

This photomicrograph shows HIV particles being released from T lymphocytes into the bloodstream.

What is HIV?

HIV is a single strand of genetic material surrounded by a protein coat. It enters a **host cell** and uses parts of the host cell to make copies of its genetic material and assemble new protein coats. The new viruses that have been made then leave the host cell and circulate in the blood to infect other host cells. This process is the same as that used by other viruses. HIV is different because the host cells it targets are T **lymphocytes** (T-cells). As the number of virus particles in the body increases, the number of T-cells slowly decreases, and the person's immune system becomes less efficient.

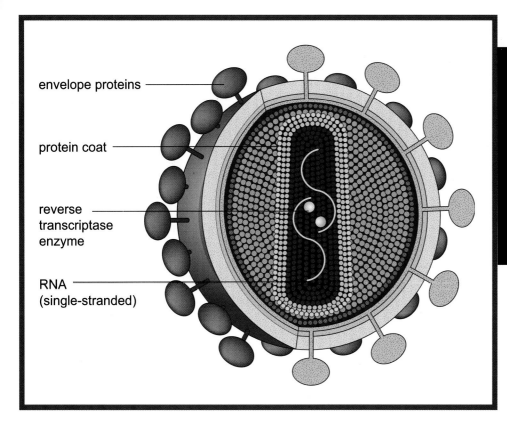

envelope proteins

protein coat

reverse
transcriptase
enzyme

RNA
(single-stranded)

HIV viruses are so small that hundreds of thousands could fit on the head of a pin!

HIV-positive

People with HIV are said to be HIV-positive. This means that a blood test has shown there are **antibodies** to the HIV virus circulating in the person's blood. Some people with HIV infection may have no symptoms at all. Others suffer from an illness similar to flu, with joint pain, a sore throat, and swollen **lymph nodes.** It can take several years for HIV to destroy enough T-cells to make the person immunodeficient but, finally, the immune system collapses. The person suffers from one infection after another. Eventually, many people with AIDS die from a common infection that their bodies cannot fight.

Treatment

At present, there is no cure for AIDS, and no **vaccine** is available. However, there are two groups of drugs that can help keep people with HIV well:

- drugs that interfere with the reproduction of the virus's **genetic** material
- drugs that interfere with the production of the **protein** coats.

Most people with HIV benefit from a triple therapy, which consists of two drugs to block genetic-material reproduction and one drug to block protein-coat production. This treatment leads to a reduction in the number of virus particles and an increase in the number of healthy T-cells. The triple therapy also seems to delay the progress from HIV infection to AIDS. The drugs involved are extremely expensive, however, and many people cannot tolerate their harsh side effects.

TRANSPLANTS AND REJECTION

At one time, when a vital organ such as the heart or lungs became damaged or diseased, a patient faced certain death. Nowadays, in many cases, advances in transplant techniques allow doctors to replace the failing organ with a healthy one donated from another person. This gives the patient the chance of a new life.

Transplants are needed to provide patients with new organs or tissues to replace their own, which are damaged or diseased. The organs most commonly transplanted are hearts, lungs, livers, and kidneys. Donated organs may come from people who have died in a traffic accident, for example, or, in the case of kidneys, from close family members, who may donate one of their own kidneys to save a relative. **Bone marrow** transplants within families are also common.

A patient's body can reject transplanted organs. This means that the immune system of the person receiving the organ (the host) recognizes **antigens** on the surface of the transplanted organ as non-self and reacts against it.

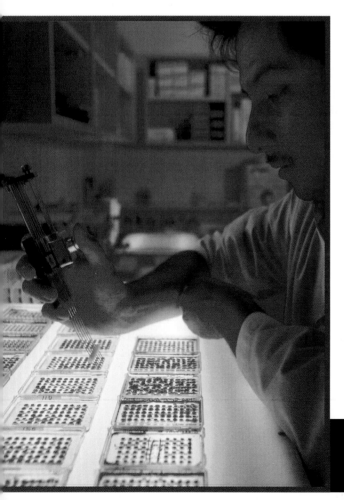

Tissue type

Every person has a set of antigens on every cell of the body, determined by the **genetic** material. There are many different possible antigens, and they can be found together in an almost infinite variety of combinations. Your own personal set of antigens is called your **tissue type.**

The risk of **rejection** is reduced if the tissue type of the transplanted organ is similar to that of the host. Ideally, the tissue types of transplant and host would be identical, but this is rarely ever possible. Before a transplant is performed, scientists perform tissue-typing tests to check that the transplant and host are not too different.

This scientist is testing the tissue type of a patient.

National and international databanks keep records of tissue types of patients and potential donors. This means that when a donor organ becomes available, it can be quickly matched with a suitable patient.

Stem cell transplants

Stem cells can be transplanted instead of bone marrow. Stem cells are the cells from which all blood cells develop. Some stem cells circulate in the blood and can be collected by a process called apheresis. Stem cell transplants can be from a donor, or a patient's own healthy stem cells can be collected and stored before radiotherapy or chemotherapy treatment begins. When the treatment is complete, his or her own stem cells can be transplanted back to restore normal bone marrow function.

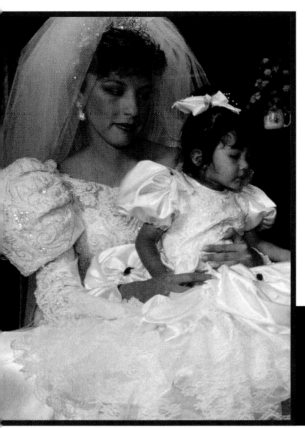

This girl has had a successful bone marrow transplant to cure her leukemia. Bone marrow was donated by her younger sister.

Suitable donors

Family members often have very similar tissue types and can, therefore, often provide tissue for transplantation. Bone marrow transplants between brother and sister or parent and child are common and are often successful in treating diseases such as leukemia.

To reduce the risk of a transplant being rejected, the patient is usually given **immunosuppressant** drugs. These turn off the immune system so that it cannot attack the transplant.

In some cases of bone marrow transplant, the opposite to transplant rejection can occur. **Lymphocytes** from the transplanted bone marrow recognize the host's body as non-self and begin to attack it. This is called a graft-versus-host reaction (GVH). It can be treated with **steroids** or immunosuppressant drugs.

Infectious mononucleosis

This illness is often known as glandular fever. It is caused by the Epstein-Barr **virus** and is most common in teenagers and young adults. Girls are three times more likely to suffer from it than boys.

The virus particles multiply in B **lymphocytes** (B-cells) in lymphatic tissue and spread into the bloodstream. The infection usually causes fever, tiredness, sore throat, and headache. The **lymph nodes** in the neck are often swollen, and there may be liver problems. Blood tests show a very high number of lymphocytes in the blood. There is no cure for the illness, but it usually lasts just a few weeks and does not have long-term effects.

In adults, the virus cannot be passed from one person to another by casual contact. In children and teenagers, it can be passed during close contact, such as by kissing or sharing drinking glasses.

Chronic fatigue syndrome

This illness has different names in different places. In Japan, it is known as low natural killer cell syndrome. In Britain it is called

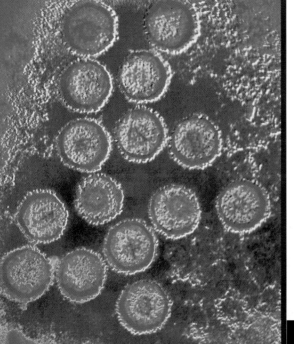

myalgic encephalomyelitis, usually shortened to ME, or post-viral syndrome. In the United States, it is referred to as chronic fatigue syndrome (CFS).

Symptoms

People with CFS have flu-like symptoms and suffer from extreme tiredness. There are often other symptoms, such as hair loss, joint and muscle pain, depression, and insomnia. The illness may last for several months, after which the person is fully well again. Some people find they have a recurrence after a few years. In other people, the illness lasts for many years without significant improvement.

This electronmicrograph shows Epstein-Barr viruses, responsible for infectious mononucleosis.

Causes

The exact cause of CFS is unknown. Scientists think that it may be linked to a viral infection, but there also seem to be some **genetic** factors that make some people more susceptible to it than others. Extreme stress is thought to play a part in the development of the illness, and there may be some dietary links.

The illness initially weakens the patient's immune system, allowing infections to develop. Some T lymphocytes seem to respond by overreacting, while others underreact. There is no cure for CFS, but many patients do improve after a period of resting and avoiding unnecessary stress.

Malignant diseases

Cells of the **lymphatic system** and immune system can undergo changes that transform them from normal cells into cancer cells.

Lymphomas are cancers of the lymphatic system. Hodgkin's disease is a lymphoma that most commonly affects teenagers and young adults. It begins in lymphoid tissue, often in the lymph nodes of the neck. These swell, and other lymph nodes become involved. The cause of Hodgkin's disease is unknown, but it is usually completely curable by a combination of radiotherapy and chemotherapy.

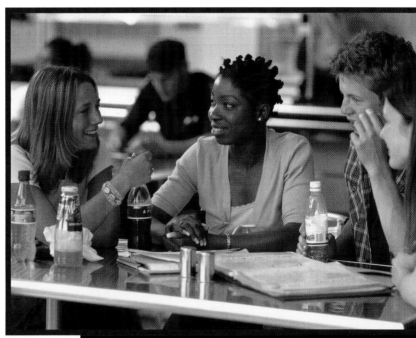

Hodgkin's disease can occur in both adults and children, and about 10 to 15 percent of all cases occur in children under 16 years old.

Leukemia

Leukemias are cancers of the blood and can arise in **bone marrow** or lymphatic tissue. There are several different forms of leukemia, but they are all caused by white blood cells failing to mature properly. These abnormal cells cannot fight infections. So many of them are produced that they eventually clog up the system, preventing the production of normal blood cells. Many leukemias are curable with radiotherapy, chemotherapy, and bone marrow transplants.

WHAT CAN GO WRONG WITH THE IMMUNE SYSTEM?

This book has explained the different parts of the immune system, why they are important, and how they can be damaged by injury and illness. This table summarizes some of the problems that can affect the immune system. It also gives information about how each problem can be treated.

Many of the problems below can be avoided or prevented by maintaining a healthy lifestyle. Getting regular exercise and plenty of rest are important, as is eating a balanced diet. This is especially important in your teenage years, when your body is still developing. The table tells you some of the ways you can prevent injury and illness.

Remember, if you think something is wrong with your body, you should always talk to a trained medical professional, such as a doctor or your school nurse. Regular medical checkups are an important part of maintaining a healthy body.

Illness or injury	Cause	Symptoms	Prevention	Treatment
allergic reaction	exposure to something to which the immune system has become hypersensitive	various, including skin rash, sickness, diarrhea, breathing difficulty, and a runny nose	avoid exposure to the triggering substance	depends on the cause, but antihistamines may help in many cases
chronic fatigue syndrome	unknown, but may be linked to stress, diet, and **viral** infection	extreme tiredness, flu-like symptoms, depression, joint and muscle pains	maintain a healthy lifestyle, with a balanced diet, and avoid stress where possible	no cure yet, but rest, reduction of stress, and a restricted diet can help in many cases
infectious mononucleosis	infection by Epstein-Barr virus	fever, tiredness, sore throat, headache, and swollen **lymph nodes**	avoid infection by the virus, for example, by not sharing drinking glasses	no cure, but with rest, recovery is usually within a few weeks
tonsillitis	infection of the tonsils, usually by **bacteria,** sometimes by a virus	sore throat, difficulty swallowing, earache, high temperature, and swollen nodes	maintain a healthy lifestyle, with a balanced diet and a good standard of hygiene	**antibiotics** to combat bacterial infection; in severe cases, tonsils may be surgically removed

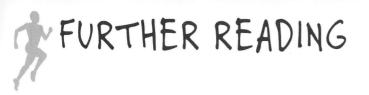

FURTHER READING

Derkins, Susie. *The Immune System.* New York: Rosen, 2001.

Gedatus, Gustav Mark. *HIV and AIDS.* Mankato, Minn.: Capstone, 1999.

McPhee, Andrew T. *AIDS.* Danbury, Conn.: Scholastic, 2001.

Monroe, Judy. *Allergies.* Mankato: Minn.: Capstone, 2001.

Silverstein, Alvin. *Allergies.* Danbury, Conn.: Scholastic, 2000.

GLOSSARY

allergic reaction reaction by the body to an antigen to which it is sensitive, such as the runny nose and sore eyes of people with hay fever when exposed to pollens

allergy sensitivity to something

anaphylactic shock acute response to an antigen that must be treated as an emergency

antibiotic drug used to fight infections. Antibiotics destroy microbes such as bacteria or fungi, but are not effective against viruses.

antibody chemical made by lymphocytes that binds to a specific antigen

antigen substance that provokes a response by the immune system

autoimmunity condition where the immune system recognizes part of the body as non-self and begins to attack it

bacterium microbe that can be useful or can cause disease

bone marrow part of the bone where white blood cells are produced

cytoplasm part of a cell outside the nucleus but inside the cell membrane

enzyme protein that helps a chemical reaction to occur

genetic having to do with passing characteristics from one generation to the next

hemophilia hereditary condition in which blood does not clot properly

histamine chemical released when tissue is damaged

host cell cell in which a virus makes more copies of itself

immunodeficiency condition in which some or all components of the immune system are missing

immunosuppression condition in which the immune system is unable to operate efficiently

inflammatory response nonspecific response to an antigen

intestine part of the digestive system

lymph clear, colorless liquid that flows through the lymphatic system

lymph node swelling on a lymph duct, where some white blood cells are made and some immune responses take place

lymphatic system system of drainage vessels, also involved in the body's immune responses

lymphocyte white blood cell that is involved in specific responses to antigens

macrophage specialized phagocyte that engulfs and destroys foreign material

membrane thin covering layer of tissue

microbe living organism, such as a bacterium, that can be seen only with a microscope

microorganism living thing only visible under a microscope

mucus sticky, slimy fluid that provides lubrication inside many organs and vessels

neutrophil specialized phagocyte

phagocyte white blood cell that engulfs microbes and cell debris

phagocytosis process of engulfing and destroying microbes and cell debris

platelet particle involved in blood clotting

protein complex chemical that is a component of many of the body's structures

rejection process by which transplanted tissue is recognized as non-self and attacked by the immune system

serum liquid part of blood

spleen largest organ in the lymphatic system

stem cell cell from which all white blood cells develop

steroid human-made drug that is similar to some chemicals found naturally in the body

thymus part of the lymphatic system where T lymphocytes mature

tissue type set of antigens on the surface of the body's cells

vaccine protection against a disease by injection of dead or weakened antigen

virus microbe that uses the body's own cells to make copies of itself; viral means something related to or caused by a virus

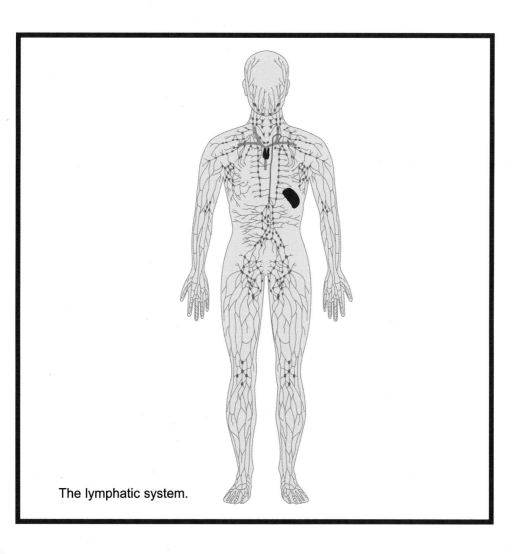

The lymphatic system.

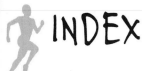

INDEX